PREMENSTRUAL SYNDROME AND ITS MANAGEMENT WITH HERBS

By
Prof. (Dr.) Kundan Singh Bora

University Institute of Pharma Sciences
Chandigarh University, Gharuan, Mohali,
Punjab-140413, INDIA.

TABLE OF CONTENT		
Sr. No.	Content	Page no.
1	Introduction	3-5
2	The reasons behind premenstrual syndrome	6-7
3	Classification of premenstrual syndrome	8-9
4	Use of modern medication	10-11
5	Management of PMS with herbs	12-18
6	Future Prospective	19-20
7	References	21-25

1. INTRODUCTION

Women, in reproductive stages goes through various emotional and physical manifestations. These symptoms experienced by women are unified under Premenstrual Syndrome (PMS). PMS comprise of wide variety of signs and symptoms before or after menstrual cycle. This includes fatigue, food craving, mood swings, irritability and depression. Breast tenderness and bloating may be experience during menstrual cycle and menopause. On an average, 5 to 8 % women suffer with moderate to severe prodomes that may associate with substantial distress and functional impairment. These signs and symptoms were prior named as premenstrual tension (PMT) [1] or premenstrual syndrome (PMS) [2]. The specific cause of PMS is still not known yet but fluctuating hormone level is one of the indication. Here is list of possible signs and symptoms faced by women during menstruation or menopause. (Note: individual women may face both or sometimes particular symptom severely, in such case, consultation with physician is preferable). Potential emotional and physical symptoms are summarized in table 1.

Table 1: Potential Emotional and Physical Symptoms

Emotional Signs and Symptoms	Physical Signs and Symptoms
Tension or anxiety	Joint or muscle pain
Depressed mood	Headache
Crying spells	Fatigue
Mood swings and irritability or anger	Weight gain related to fluid retention
Appetite changes and food cravings	Abdominal bloating
Trouble falling asleep (insomnia)	Breast tenderness
Social withdrawal	Acne flare-ups

Poor concentration	Constipation or diarrhoea
Change in libido	Alcohol intolerance

The above symptoms may be flexible within few days and 2 weeks. Symptoms gets often prompt and unfavourable 6 days before and may be at peak stage 2 days before menstruation starts [4, 5]. Irritability, angry mood and food cravings are most complaints that are seen before other symptoms arrival. It has also been encountered that some face emotional stress severely that disturbs daily life. However, be any symptom, they should or gets vanish in four to five days as menstruation period is initiated.

Premenstrual dysphoric disorder (PMDD) is another condition in which women faces disabling symptoms every month.

2. THE REASONS BEHIND PREMENSTRUAL SYNDROME!

The exact cause for the PMS is unclear but several theories are proposed by researchers to understand the cause for the PMS. It includes excessive estrogen, progesterone deficiency, elevated prolactin, increased aldosterone, nutritional inefficiencies, and various psychologic factors [11-14]. Stress is additionally one of the main reasons for PMS [15]. PMS may also be because of interactions between ovarian hormones, endogenous opioid peptides, neurotransmitters, prostaglandins, and therefore the circadian, peripheral, autonomic, and endocrine systems [22,21,16-18]. Obesity also results in PMS. One hypothesis also suggests that PMS may be because of an aberration in blood viscosity and red blood corpuscle hydration during the menstrual cycle [19].

The imbalance of estrogen and progesterone could also be because of a disruption of the conventional feedback systems that control the hypothalamus-pituitary-ovary axis or to a dysfunction of anybody of those glands (most commonly the ovaries). This is commonly considered to point to a deficiency or failure of the corpus luteum. It may also be that the ovaries are functioning fine, but hepatic metabolism and excretion of estrogens are impaired.

Elevated prolactin levels imply a degree of pituitary imbalance or dysfunction, especially a scarcity of sensitivity to the standard inhibitory messages. Increased levels of aldosterone, like FSH, leads to a degree of pituitary dysfunction and cause insensitivity to a rising water content of the body [20]. Stress also affects the hormone production and stimulates the secretion of a variety of other hormones that interfere with the sex hormones: adrenocorticotropic hormone (ACTH), cortisol, the catecholamines such as epinephrine, and norepinephrine, and aldosterone, a corticosteroid that causes retention in renal sodium [15].

3. CLASSIFICATION OF PREMENSTRUAL SYNDROME

PMS is assessed into 4 subgroups, each with specific symptoms, hormonal pictures and metabolic abnormalities.

PMS A: A more than estrogen relative to progesterone leads to PMS A. The ratio and levels of certain neurotransmitters are going to be altered in brain by estrogen. Specifically, estrogen raises levels of adrenalin, noradrenaline and serotonin and reduces levels of dopamine and phenylethylamine. This brain stimulation brings about the symptoms of anxiety, nervous tension and mood swings.

PMS C: Prostaglandin imbalance, Hypoglycaemia and Magnesium deficiency leads to PMS C [23]. It is characterized by a rise in appetite, looking for simple carbohydrates (breads, sugars, grains, snack foods), fluctuations in blood glucose, fatigue, headaches, dizziness or fainting [24].

PMS D: A more than progesterone relative to estrogen leads to PMS D, the progesterone acts on the brain as a depressant. It may also be aggravated by the low estrogen levels which lead to the breakdown of mood-enhancing neurotransmitters.

PMS H: PMS H is caused by stress, low magnesium and high estrogen, which disrupt the traditional aldosterone and involves the symptom like water retention, abdominal bloating, breast tenderness, and weight gain [25-26]

4. USE OF MODERN MEDICATION

PMS may interfere in daily activities and create stressful condition in working hours of certain women. To rule out this issue, there are number of medications may or may not be prescribed by physician. There are certain recommended medications such as antidepressants, Non-steroidal Anti-Inflammatory Drugs (NSAIDs) and hormonal contraceptives which helps in reducing symptoms caused during PMS.

Antidepressants like Selective Serotonin Reuptake Inhibitors (SSRI) are mostly prescribed and recommended in PMS. It is first line treatment for PMDD and PMS. Already known that hormonal imbalance leads to mood swings, anxiety and anger. Serotonin is responsible for stabilizing mood and calming effects, resulting use of SSRIs increase the concentration of serotonin. Fluoxetine, Paroxetine and Sertraline are some popular antidepressants [9]. Side effects may experience by individual are nausea, fatigue, weight gain, blurred vision and constipation.

Non-steroidal Anti-Inflammatory Drugs (NSAIDs) are agents having capability to decrease the menstrual cramps and breast tenderness. Ibuprofen and naproxen sodium are preferred NSAIDs. On administration of NSAIDs ingestion, dizziness, stomach ulcers and allergic reaction may occur. That's why, always recommended to use after consulting physician.

Diuretics and hormonal contraceptives are used because of insufficient intake of salt and lack of exercise and to terminate ovulation. Spironolactone is majorly used in PMS as diuretics. Side effects like dehydration, impotence and headaches may be noticed. Hormonal contraceptive may include use of vitamin B_6 supplementation. Calcium and magnesium intake is also preferred along with exercise [10]. Hormonal contraceptives side effects accounts for sore breasts, decreased sexual desire, weight gain and acne.

5. MANAGEMENT OF PMS WITH HERBS

Hamidpour R and Rashan L [8] studied the therapeutic effects of some herbal drugs on PMS. They togtherly give psychological, physical and behavioural effect to reduce symptoms during PMS.

According to them, 85% of women face premenstrual syndrome every month during their menstruation. Management of PMS primarily depends on signs and symptoms and their severity. Women facing premenstrual dysphoric disorder (PMDD) should consult physician for getting relief immediately. There are various drugs available in market on prescription. Antidepressant, diuretics, anti-inflammatories, and hormone contraceptives are mostly used in PMS but they may cause side effects. Use of herbal medicines is preferred by many women as they have least side effects, easily available and are suitable. One of the herbal medication is "Pain 6" which is combination of six herbs naturally occurring in nature. It is manufactured by "Pars Biosciences".

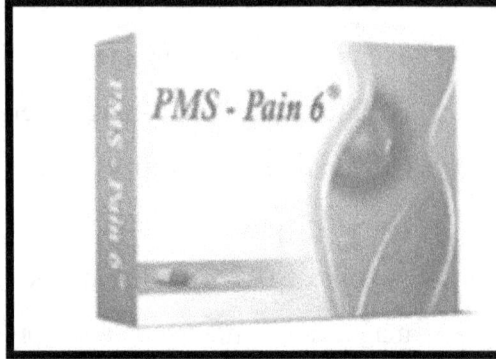

- *Salvia officinalis* (sage)

- *Foeniculum vulgare* (fennel)
- *Urtica diodica* (nettle)
- *Taraxacum officinale* (dandelion)
- *Petroselinum crispum* (parsley)
- *Equistum arvense* (horsetail)

Herbal formulations are used from ancient times for management of problems associated with menstruation and menopause. There are some herbs listed in table 2 which are reported to be useful to reduce symptoms of PMS. These herbs can be consumed with tea, water and honey. They are available in the form of both, powder and tonic [6, 7].

Table 2: Herbs used in PMS

Symptom	Name of the Herb	Action
Menopausal symptoms	Black cohosh	Bind estrogen receptor, inhibits Luteinizing Hormone secretion and

		nonreceptormediated action
Premenstrual syndrome	Chaste tree fruit	Alters Follicular stimulating hormone and Luteinizing Hormone levels; increases progesterone levels
Sleep disturbances	Lemon balm	Tranquilizer/ sedative
Impaired concentration	Ginkgo	Stimulates circulation and oxygen flow
Fatigue, loss of concentration	Ginseng	Uterine Stimulant
Anxiety, Insomnia	Passion flower	Sedative
Depression	St. John's wort	Antidepressant

Nervousness	Valerian	Sedative
Women's discomforts	Dong quai	Uterus stimulant, analgesic
Reduces LDL cholesterol	Flax seed	Phytoestrogen
Menopausal symptoms	Red clover	Phytoestrogen
PMS & Menopausal symptoms	Fennel & Fenugreek	Phytoestrogen and rich in calcium
Menopausal symptoms	Wild Yam	Phytoestrogen
Muscular cramps	Palm jaggery	Rich in Vitamin B, zinc, & Magnesium

PMS is a broad group of symptoms, although every women facing PMS suffer some specifc symptoms. Also there's not a single herb which can be used as silver bullet for all symptoms. Hence, it is best to use one or more herb according to the symptoms facing during PMS. Most of women utlilize this formula and is helpful.

Digestive Problems: Gas, nausea, diarrhea, constipation and heartburn are categrized under digestive issues. In this case, culinary herbs help to tackle with symptoms. Licorice, ginger, mint, lemon and honey are potential soothing agents in digestive problems. These herbs are ingredient of almost every ayurvedic medicines used in gastrointenstinal disorders. Another herb is *Poria sclerotium,* a fungus useful in digestive function.

Emotional Problems: Mood swings, feeling down, irritability and anxiety fall under emotional problems. Here, mood elevating herbs are promising remedies. Peony root, Cyperus rhizome and bupleurum are popular herbs used in PMS. Valerian choice of herb for sleeplessness, irritability and tension.

Cramps, headaches, breast tenderness and pain: For these type of symptoms, herbs possessing anti-inflammatory competency are used. Turmeric, active ingredient curcumin is widely used for chronic pain and spams. Many times, Dong quai root is prescribed for cramps and headaches. For detoxification of liver function, Chinese skullcap, an anti-inflammatory herb is beneficial.

According to a study, fennel is having efficacy as mefenamic acid, mostly prescribed in period pain. Fennel is widely studied for its effectiveness over dysmenorrhea or severe pain. Most of people use, fennel as mouth refreshing agent to prevent nausea and fatigue. Likewise, cinnamon is used to decrease rid of pain and cramping. Its therapeutic efficacy is nearly same as Ibuprofen, a NSAID. Resembling to fennel, cinnamon is also used to prevent and avoid nausea and vomiting during PMS and menstruation.

Ginger root, commonly known as "adrak" is always available in kitchen. Ginger is has a broad therapeutic range, useful in pain, headache, gastrointestinal tract disorders, low back pain, joint pain and muscle weakness. It has potency similar to ibuprofen and mefenamic acid. There are many home remedies for PMS, which have low or no side effects as compared to modern medication.

6. FUTURE PROSPECTIVE

PMS or PMDD is suffered by most of women during menstruation and menopause. They are triggered by cyclic changes in hormones, and chemical alteration in brain. It is known that serotonin, a neurotransmitter responsible for mood changes plays a vital role in PMS. To tackle with the symptoms causes during menstruation and menopause, women seeks to physician for medication. Many allopathic medicines are available at pharmacy which help and provide instant relief from pain. Along with it, many side effects are experienced by users which creates another issue for most of women. To avoid these unexpected effects associated with modern medications, herbal formulations are utilized widely. Herbal medicines are now preferred over allopathic medication as they possess least or no side effects. Herbs like ginger root, cinnamon, and ginseng are commonly available in home kitchen. They can be used to get relief from nausea and vomiting instantly. Apart from it, general awareness campaign should be carried out to make aware women regarding PMS and its management. A lot research is still needed in discovering various herbs useful in PMS and menopause.

7. REFERENCES

1. Frank R. The hormonal causes of premenstrual tension. Arch Neurol Psychiatry 1931; 26: 1053–57.

2. Greene R, Dalton K. The premenstrual syndrome. BMJ 1953; 1: 1007–14

3. Premenstrual syndrome (PMS) Signs and Symptoms by Mayoclinic Organization.

Premenstrual syndrome (PMS) - Symptoms and causes - Mayo Clinic

4. Pearlstein T, Yonkers K, Fayyad R, Gillespie J. Pretreatment pattern of symptom expression in premenstrual dsyphoric disorder. J Aff ect Disord 2005; 85: 275–82.

5. Meaden PM, Hartlage SA, Cook-Kerr J. Timing and severity of symptoms associated with the menstrual cycle in a community-based sample in the Midwestern United States. Psychiatr Res 2005; 134: 27–36.

6. Holly Bellebuono..November, An Herbalist's Guide to Formulary: The Art and Science of Creating Effective Herbal Remedies. Concious Lifestyle Magazine.2012. www.cociouslifestylemag.org

7. Lowdermilk, &Perry . "Maternity and Women's Health care". (8thed.).2008. New York : Mosby company.

8. Hamidpour R, Rashan L (2017) An Herbal Preparation that Relieves Symptoms of Premenstrual Syndrome. Transl Biomed Vol 8 Iss 3: 126. doi:10.21767/2172-0479.1000126

9. Freeman EW, Rickels K, Sondheimer SJ, Polansky M. Differential Response to Antidepressants in Women With Premenstrual Syndrome/Premenstrual Dysphoric Disorder: A Randomized Controlled Trial. Arch Gen Psychiatry. 1999;56(10):932–939. doi:10.1001/archpsyc.56.10.932

10. Andrea Rapkin, A review of treatment of premenstrual syndrome & premenstrual dysphoric disorder, Psychoneuroendocrinology, Volume 28, Supplement 3, 2003, Pages 39-53, ISSN 0306-4530, https://doi.org/10.1016/S0306-4530(03)00096-9.

11. Wolinsky I and Klimis-Tavantzis D: editors. Nutritional Concerns of Women. New York: CRC Press; 1996.

12. 1223. Smith S and Schiff I: The premenstrual syndrome-diagnosis and management. FertilSteril.1989; 52: 527-43.

13. Lyon KE and Lyon MA: The premenstrual syndrome; a survey of current treatment practices. J Reprod Med. 1984; 29: 705-11.

14. Sherwood RA and Rocks BF: Magnesium and the premenstrual syndrome. Ann ClinBiochem. 1986; 23: 667-70.

15. McIntyre A. The Complete Woman's Herbal. New York: Henry Holt; 1994.

16. Mira M, Stewart PM and Abraham SF: Vitamin and trace element status in premenstrual syndrome. Am J ClinNutr.1988; 47: 636-41.

17. Abraham GE. Nutritional factors in the etiology of the premenstrual tension syndromes. J Reprod Med.1983; 28: 446-64.

18. Lee CM andLeklem JE: Blood magnesium constancy with vitamin B-6 supplementation in pre- and post-menopausal women. Ann Clin and Lab Sci.1984; 14: 151-54.
19. Simpson LO. The etiopathologies of premenstrual syndrome as a consequence of altered blood rheology: A new hypothesis. Med Hypothesis. 1988; 25(4).
20. http://medherb.com/Therapeutics/Female_-_Premenstrual_Syndrome.htm
21. Smith S and Schiff I: The premenstrual syndrome-diagnosis and management. FertilSteril.1989; 52: 527-43
22. Reid RL and Yen SSC: Premenstrual syndrome. Am J Obstet Gynecol.1981;139: 85-104.
23. http://www.toddcaldecott.com/index.php/healing/conditions/230 premenstrualsyndrome.
24. http://www.globinmed.com/index.php?option=com_content&view=article&id=77768 : Premenstrual-Syndrome-(PMS).

25. http://medherb.com/Therapeutics/Female_-_Premenstrual_Syndrome.htm.
26. http://www.globinmed.com/index.php?option=com_content&view=article&id=77768 : Premenstrual-Syndrome-(PMS) &catid=493 : p

www.ingramcontent.com/pod-product-compliance
Lightning Source LLC
Chambersburg PA
CBHW071001220526
45471CB00007B/3131

9798343058574